"Steve White's book, *When* scription of his journey with kidney disease, his struggles navigating the world of transplant, and the decision to live with dialysis as seen through the eyes of an actual patient. It is a valuable resource to others who may find themselves in this situation along with their families. It is a story of how his faith in God helped him find the strength to decide to live with the diagnosis and help others by sharing his personal testimony."
—*Denise Neal, RN. BSN, BS, CPTC, Transplant Coordinator*

"Mr. White's book describes his firsthand encounter with end-stage renal failure. His transparent, faith-filled courage throughout the past three years are a testimony to his deep faith in the Great Physician. His close walk with God and his positive attitude are an inspiration to us all."
—*Peter Hill and Joyce Hill (co-author,* The God I Know and the Relationship We Need*)*

"In his book, Steve White tells the very personal story of his medical journey and how he is thriving on the other side of significant adversity. His story will be an inspiration and comfort to many others who feel alone as they travel this unfamiliar landscape. His story is one of strength and perseverance."
—*Dr. Laura Gonzalez, M.D. Cardiologist*

"Mr. White has been a challenging but wonderful patient. He wants to know everything about everything regarding his disease and treatment, but he has also been compliant and done everything we've asked him to do. He has made great progress with his disease, and I wish I could give all my patients his attitude. His story is inextricable from his faith and contains valuable information for patients and families dealing with kidney disease."
—*Dr. Anupama Gowda, M.D. Nephrologist*

When Kidneys Fail

A Story of Faith

Steve White

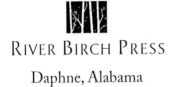

RIVER BIRCH PRESS

Daphne, Alabama

ISBN 978-1-956365-17-7 (print)
ISBN 978-1-956365-18-4 (e-book)

For Worldwide Distribution
Printed in the U.S.A.

River Birch Press
P.O. Box 868, Daphne, AL 36526

To Tonya...
And to all the other medical personnel
that work with patients suffering from kidney disease.
You go to work every day to keep me alive.

Never underestimate your value,
how much you are appreciated,
and the difference you make in my life.
I love you and I salute you!

Table of Contents

Foreword

There is no easy way to hear that one needs dialysis, and it is probably even harder to receive a cancer diagnosis. Many people think they know what they would do when faced with these kinds of life-altering events. They may have preconceived notions about what therapies they will and will not accept. But when the time comes, and one faces the terrifying truth, decisions and behavior may change.

Mr. White was faced with both of these diagnoses, compounded by a diagnosis of Covid-19, which led him to look fear in the eyes and make decisions about his care that shocked even him. His faith in the Lord carried him all along his journey, giving him strength to ultimately navigate his medical issues.

Medicine is not always straightforward, and often medical problems and situations evolve over time as new information is revealed. Through his book When Kidneys Fail – A Story of Faith, Mr. White highlights his journey through the dreaded diagnosis, ultimately taking him to the brink of death and back again.

Dr. Sarah Friend, MD
Assistant Professor of Medicine
Department of Hematology and Medical Oncology

Introduction

This book is written for people with kidney disease, their families, and their medical teams.

I learned that I had kidney disease in early 2019. By September of that year my kidney function had dropped to 30%. That started me on a medical journey that was far beyond my wildest imagination. I had to face it. I'd been dealt a bad hand and I had to deal with it.

By the fall of 2021, the journey had been just over three years, during which I faced many mental, emotional, physical, financial, and spiritual issues. It has involved family, friends, doctors, nurses, and donors (some of whom were total strangers to me). I have endured enormous stress throughout this time. All along the way I have had to make dozens of choices—and for me it included life or death!

You are going to face many of the same choices I faced. I want to tell you my story in hopes that something in my experience will help you with your journey. I'm going to share raw emotions, stressful situations, my fear, my anger, family dynamics, financial pressures, mental struggles, and the choices I faced.

I will not just share my choices, but I'll share *why* I made them, and the results those choices created for me in my journey. Hopefully this will help you make the choices best for you. Choices aren't good or bad, right or wrong; they are just choices, and you must make them. You will be offered advice (sometimes by everyone), but at the end of the day, the buck stops with you.

I consider myself to be a spiritual man with a deep faith. Along the telling of my journey, I will share with you the spiritual issues I faced, how I dealt with them, and reasons for my trust in God. I certainly realize that not every person shares my faith, nor is it my intent that you buy in to my belief system. But you do believe in something—your gut, your instincts, your intellect. Wherever or to whomever you go in times of fear and uncertainty, you will be alone with them and with your choices.

When I am scared and not sure what to do, I go to God because my trust is in Him. Psalm 57:1 says,

Have mercy on me of God, have mercy on me, for in you I take refuge. I will take refuge in the shadow of your wings until the disaster has passed.

Nahum 1:7 says it again: "The Lord is good, a refuge in times of trouble. He cares for those who trust in him."

Maybe you're not a believer. If so, consider seeking Him. Read this next verse from Psalm 9:10 very carefully, "Those who know your name will trust in you, for you, Lord, have never forsaken those who seek you." Test Him on this! "Ask and it will be given to you; seek and you shall find; knock and the door will be opened to you" (Matt. 7:7).

At the end of each chapter, you will find a section called "Takeaways," where I offer advice and the most important things to remember as you face your medical choices.

I hope the experiences I'm able to share will help you along your way. I will also offer you some advice about your medical choices. But I will tell you this—the single greatest thing that you can do for yourself on your journey is to have a good attitude about it. Kidneys don't get better, so just accept it, embrace it, and do your best with the hand you've been dealt.

All along the way, just keep in mind that God loves you, and He knows the mess you're in!

1

The Day It All Began

I had been to see my Primary Care Physician (PCP), Dr. Scott Henderson, and he noticed in my blood work that my creatinine levels had been increasing steadily over the previous year. He recommended that I see a nephrologist. Now I had no idea what a nephrologist was, but I soon learned it was a kidney doctor. Dr. Henderson referred me to Dr. Susan Hill, but she was booked solid. So I saw another doctor in that practice. The first nephrologist I ever met was Dr. Anupama Gowda, who remains my physician to this day.

Creatinine is a breakdown product of creatine phosphate from muscle and from dietary meat intake. As a waste product, creatinine is filtered out of the blood by the kidneys and removed from the body through urine. A creatinine test measures the amount of this chemical in either the blood or the urine. The normal range of creatinine in the blood is between .7–1.2mg per deciliter. Mine was over 3.0.

The level of creatinine in your blood is the primary variable used to calculate the effectiveness of your kidneys. The technical term for how well your kidneys are functioning is called the Glomerular Filtration Rate (GFR). Glomeruli are the tiny filters in the kidney that filter waste from the blood. In young healthy humans, the GFR should be 100%. It declines with age but normally never reaches a level that requires any treatment.

In September 2019 my GFR was 30. My kidneys were only functioning at 30% efficiency. I had stage four chronic kidney disease (CKD).

Treatment Plan

Dr. Gowda immediately told me to do two things: lose weight and reduce my salt intake. At the time, I weighed about 290 pounds and since I'm only six feet one inch, clinically I was considered morbidly obese. I'd never thought of myself as morbidly obese, and it really jolted me that from a medical perspective, that is exactly what I was! Reducing my salt intake was hard for me since I'm a salt freak. While I tried to do it, I'm sure it was nowhere near the degree to which she wanted.

The third component to Dr. Gowda's plan was to adjust my blood pressure medications. While diabetes is the leading cause of CKD, hypertension is the second leading cause. My blood pressure was averaging about 140/90, and while my PCP thought it was at goal, Dr. Gowda informed me that it was still way too high.

For years, the conventional wisdom among PCPs was that 140/90 was an acceptable level, and my PCP had me on blood pressure meds to keep it at that level. It probably stayed at that level for over ten years, and all that time, unbeknownst to me, my kidneys were gradually deteriorating. Through increased medication, Dr. Gowda brought my BP down to 120/75.

The idea was to lose weight, reduce salt, and lower my BP. Hopefully this would put me on a path that would allow my kidneys to function normally for the rest of my life. However, the real damage had already been done, and my kidneys were already in a steep decline. At only 30% efficiency, I was in trouble, and my kidneys were probably not going to last a lifetime. This was extremely upsetting news to me.

I had never really spent much time thinking about my own mortality, but here it was right in front of me. One tends to think one is invincible and will live forever, but suddenly that thought was now in question. I have a strong faith and no fear of death since I am assured of my eternal home in heaven, I just wasn't ready to go today!

The apostle Paul said,

"Death has been swallowed up in victory. Where, O death, is your victory? Where, O death is your sting?" The sting of death is sin and the power of sin is the law. But thanks be to God! He gives us the victory through our Lord Jesus Christ (1 Cor. 15:54-56).

I know that I belong to God. I am His. Isaiah 43:1 says, "Do not fear for I have redeemed you; I have summoned you by name; you are mine." It is important to know where you are and what you are, but to know whose you are is the greatest comfort.

Dr. Gowda then ordered a kidney biopsy because my kidney function had declined so rapidly.

Because what I had was so serious, I was encouraged to get a second opinion. I went to see Dr. Susan Hill, another local nephrologist, and she confirmed Dr. Gowda's diagnosis and treatment plan. I asked Dr. Gowda if I had hurt her feelings by getting a second opinion, and she said no. However, she did say she was surprised and thought maybe I didn't believe she had been thorough in her evaluation and diagnosis.

I did not feel that way at all, and I regret that I had made her feel that way. I am very confident in Dr. Gowda, and she is my nephrologist for the duration, whatever that may be.

Alternative Treatments

Because kidney disease doesn't get better, and the damage done is irreversible, the best anyone can do is stop further decline in kidney function. Therefore, I started doing some research on alternative treatments for kidney disease. In November 2019 I found clinical trials using stem cells at both the Mayo Clinic and the Cleveland Clinic. In the following weeks, I visited both of those facilities only to learn through their testing that my kidneys were too far gone to be eligible.

At the Cleveland Clinic in Florida, I met with a nephrologist named Dr. Rute Paixao. She is a tall woman from Brazil. I told her I had end-stage renal failure and was looking to participate in any stem cell trials they were conducting. She asked me if I was on dialysis and I told her no. She promptly informed me, "Well then, you're not at end-stage renal failure if you're not on dialysis." I thought her response was strange. She told me that all the stem cell trials were in Cleveland but that my kidney function was too low to be eligible.

While at the Mayo Clinic, I met with Dr. LaTonya Hickson, a nephrologist engaged in kidney research. I shared with her that I was not really interested in dialysis. She suggested that a kidney transplant seemed like a good option for me. A fellow doctor from Mayo, Dr. Arpita Basu, had just left and gone to work as a transplant nephrologist at Emory University, which was right in my backyard.

I reached out to Dr. Basu to inquire about the process for entering the transplant protocol. She returned my call herself. I'll never forget receiving the call on my cell phone as I was walking out of the local barbershop. Dr. Basu was very personable, answered all my questions, and spent a lot of time with me on the phone. I was scared and uncertain, but I had to decide what I wanted to do next.

Takeaways

1. *Stay on top of your numbers,* especially your creatinine. The higher your creatinine, the lower your GFR. If your GFR ever falls below 50, then go see a nephrologist at your earliest convenience. Also watch your BP and try to keep it at less than 130/75. You want to stop the decline of your kidney function as early as possible so they will last for your lifetime. And remember, bad news early is good news. Whether it's breast cancer, prostate cancer, or kidney disease, early treatment greatly increases success rates.

2. *Seek alternative treatments* like stem cells. Medical science achieves breakthroughs every day. Pray about those that might be suitable for you.

3. *When your GFR is above 20, do everything you can to keep it there.* When your GFR falls below 20, you are eligible to be referred for a kidney transplant evaluation. Your nephrologist can facilitate a referral to a transplant center. If that happens, start the transplant testing protocol right away at the closest transplant facility. You have time before dialysis will be required (usually when GFR gets to 10 or lower). Transplants are more successful if the patient has never been on dialysis.

4. *Start soliciting donors.* You can't have too many. I had sixteen but ended up with only one, who wasn't even my blood type.

5. *Never give up hope.* "Now faith is confidence in what we hope for and assurance about what we do not see" (Heb. 11:1). The apostle Peter said, "Through him you believe in God, who raised him from the dead and glorified him, and so your faith and hope are in God" (1 Pet. 1:21).

2

To Transplant or Not To Transplant

The transplant decision was looming large and needed to be made very soon. We were approaching the holiday season of 2019, and Thanksgiving and Christmas were right around the corner. Meanwhile, Dr. Gowda had some further tests she wanted to run on me. She wanted to do a biopsy of my kidney to determine the specific kidney disease I had. She also wanted to do a twenty-four-hour urine collection test, which she felt was a better gauge of kidney function.

Because I anticipated a tremendous medical expense involved, I started a GoFundMe account as well as posted my need on Facebook, sending it to my closest friends. I was absolutely astounded by the incredible response I received. I took the account down within thirty days when donations had met my goal, which helped with the expenses of visiting the Mayo and Cleveland Clinics. I had no idea what future expenses I would face. I knew the surgeries would be expensive, and the immunosuppressant drugs were also projected to be significant.

I should also note at this point that I had no real symptoms that anything was wrong. In many patients, like me, they don't develop signs or symptoms until late stages, when GFR is below 10-15. In advanced stages, a patient can develop:

- Nausea
- Vomiting
- Loss of appetite
- Fatigue and weakness
- Sleep problems
- Urinating less
- Decreased mental sharpness
- Muscle cramps
- Swelling of the feet or ankles
- Dry, itchy skin
- Labile blood pressure
- Shortness of breath
- Chest pain (if fluid builds around the heart lining)

Other than some trouble sleeping and high BP, I had none of these symptoms. That's the tricky part because each of these symptoms is easily attributable to other causes.

Then off I went to get a kidney biopsy. I went to Northside Hospital for the procedure because they used a specific pathology company in Arkansas that specializes in kidney pathology, which Dr. Gowda preferred. There are many specific kidney diseases, such as the following:

- Nephrotic Syndrome
- Nephritis
- Autoimmune issues
- Sclerotic diseases (scarring)

The pathology of my kidney biopsy showed Dr. Gowda

that I had Nephrotic Syndrome and that I also had an abnormal monoclonal protein in the kidney that was an alarm bell for her. Multiple myeloma was a possibility, and she wanted me to go see a hematology oncologist, Dr. Sarah Friend. The thought of some type of cancer was terrifying to me. I was anxious to see Dr. Friend.

Dr. Friend is a very personable and petite lady. She is also very young. My first thought was that on her next birthday she would probably be getting her driver's license.

In fact, most of my doctors are younger than my children. What Dr. Friend lacked in size and stature, however, she more than made up for in intellect and professionalism. She ordered several more tests:

- A body survey (x-ray of the entire body)
- A positron emission tomography (PET) scan
- A bone marrow biopsy

From what I recall of the end result, they found some B-cell monoclonal lymphocytes that weren't of great concern to Dr. Friend. No multiple myeloma was detected, and she sent me back to Dr. Gowda. (Later, Denise Neal, my transplant coordinator, remembered the bone marrow biopsy as being somewhat inconclusive.) In any case, Dr. Friend was unconcerned about the findings, so the treatment plan remained lose weight, reduce salt, and keep my blood pressure low. And that's what I did through the Christmas holidays of 2019.

While I was greatly relieved that I had no imminent cancer concerns, I knew my kidney function was deteriorating rapidly, and I needed to do something soon.

I always considered a kidney transplant to be a much better option than dialysis for me. I have an advance directive that says I do not want a feeding tube or a respirator to be kept alive. My wife, Sherrie, has a medical power of attorney, and she knows my preferences. Dialysis always seemed to be an extension of that thinking. If you don't want to be kept alive by a feeding tube or respirator, why is it okay to be kept alive by a dialysis machine? I struggled with what God thought about that. Fifty years ago, it wouldn't have been an option. Two hundred years ago crossing the country in covered wagon, I would have been a dead man walking. I was still wrestling with what God thought about it.

Then I was reminded of the story of when God told Abraham to sacrifice his own son, Isaac, on the altar. Abraham never hesitated. When Isaac questioned Abraham about where the sacrificial lamb was, Abraham replied, "God himself will provide the lamb for the burnt offering, my son" (Gen. 22:8). Just as Abraham was about to plunge the knife into Isaac on the altar, God stopped him. God knew then how much Abraham trusted and believed in God.

I began to feel the same way about a kidney. I decided to trust God to provide a kidney for me, and I further believed that dialysis was God's provision for treating kidney disease. Yes, I was being kept alive by a machine, but God had something left for me to do.

My decision wasn't something that needed to be answered that day. In early January 2020, though, my GFR officially fell below 20%, and I became eligible to get on the National Kidney Foundation transplant list. I called Dr. Basu and told her I wanted to begin the transplant testing protocol at Emory.

I had no idea the magnitude of the process would be so onerous and time-consuming. And the wait-time to get a deceased donor in Georgia is still around seven or eight years.

Unless I found a matching donor of my own, I was going to be faced with dialysis because my kidneys were in no way going to last me another seven or eight years.

Takeaways

1. *Find out what your insurance covers* regarding treatment and transplants. If it is not enough to cover the expenses, start fundraising opportunities. Start a GoFundMe account and explore Facebook, as it also has some fundraising capabilities. Contact all your friends and let them know what is happening. Also, contact your church and get them involved.

2. *Get blood work done early and often* and keep a close watch on creatinine. Also keep your BP low and lose weight if your doctor advises.

3. *Listen to your nephrologist,* who will run some tests to determine your exact diagnosis. If the test results suggest seeing other specialists (as mine did), then do it right away.

4. *Get a medical power of attorney,* someone who will make medical decisions for you if you are unresponsive. Choose a person you trust, who knows what you want—and most importantly—who you are certain will carry them out as you wish. A close loved one may know that you want no heroics, but in desperation may not be able to do it.

5. *I was opposed to dialysis. You shouldn't be.* Many people are ineligible for a transplant for various reasons, and dialysis is a viable alternative.

6. The testing to be cleared to receive a kidney transplant is arduous and time-consuming. *Know that and be patient.*

7. *Find out the wait time for a deceased donor* in your state. In Georgia, it is currently seven years.

8. *Start soliciting donors* as soon as you decide to get tested for transplant. The donors must also be cleared, and they have their own medical hoops to jump through. They can start the process online. Contact friends, church social groups, and social media. I've known people to take out a billboard and signs on a bus!

3

Trying To Get Cleared

Dr. Basu put me in touch with the Emory Transplant facility, specifically the kidney transplant unit. I was assigned a transplant coordinator named Denise Neal, an RN whose job was to shepherd me through all the necessary testing and to schedule meetings with all the doctors and medical staff that I needed to meet.

I was assigned to Denise because of my doctor's area code. All nephrologists in area code 404 were assigned to Denise. Denise was very professional and all-business. She didn't seem to want much social interaction, which disappointed me, but I knew she would be diligent with my case. Later I learned that she was a big Georgia football fan, and we still exchange emails to this day about our Dawgs!

Denise told me she viewed me as very engaged and proactive. She observed that I reached out to others to find common ground (our beloved Dawgs), which made me a real person, not just a case number. The caseload of transplant coordinators is enormous, making it challenging to connect with each patient individually. So, as the patient, you need to be proactive in reaching out to them.

Denise informed me that I would be meeting with the following people:

- A transplant nephrologist
- A transplant surgeon
- A cardiologist
- A nutritionist
- A social worker
- A financial planner (to make sure I could pay)
- A psychologist
- A radiologist

And that I would have the following tests:
- An electrocardiogram (EKG)
- An electroencephalogram (EEG)
- A nuclear stress test
- An echocardiogram (ECHO)
- A computerized tomography (CT) scan
- A magnetic resonance imaging (MRI)
- Chest x-ray
- Blood chemistry evaluation
- Twenty-four-hour urine collection and evaluation

All in all, the process seemed rigorous and thorough, and it certainly seemed to cover all the medical bases to ascertain whether I was going to be cleared to receive a kidney transplant. Little did I know that the process was going to take five more months to complete. The tests were scheduled one at a time. For example, the MRI was not scheduled until the nuclear stress test was complete. When the nuclear stress test was complete, the wait time to get on the MRI schedule was three weeks. This was the process for five months, testing and meeting with doctors and transplant staff.

God was teaching me patience. As Paul said, "Hope that is seen is no hope at all. Who hopes for what they already have? But if we hope for what we do not yet have, we wait for it patiently" (Rom. 8:24-25).

Simultaneous to my testing to get cleared to receive a kidney, my potential donors were able to start the process of determining whether or not they were a potential donor. Sixteen people offered me a kidney, and later I will tell you about each one. The donors had a process of their own to go through. The online questionnaire was able to eliminate some people right off the bat. Some of the reasons to be eliminated include excess weight, chronic disorders, etc.

One surprise to me was that age was not a criterion for elimination. Eighteen was the earliest age to be a donor, but there is no upper age limit. Once the donor cleared the online exam, they were asked to submit a blood and urine sample to the transplant donor team. The donor went to a lab to have this done and waited for further feedback.

Once they determine that a donor is a matching blood type, they begin a series of tests that the donor can complete with their doctor without having to come to Emory for those tests. These tests might be an EKG, mammogram, chest x-ray, etc. Once a donor clears all those tests, they are invited to Emory for final testing and approval to become a donor.

One part of the donor process is called the Kidney Paired Exchange Program. This allows a donor who is not your blood type to remain in the donor program on a Kidney Paired Exchange basis. What that means is that my donor can give their kidney to another recipient that matches their blood type, and that recipient's donor who matches me can give me their kidney. So, if a recipient in California matches my donor, and their donor matches me, they do all four surgeries on the same day. Incredible!

The two donors have their surgeries, and the organs are then flown to the recipients (passing in the air). The transplants are done only hours after the live organs arrive.

Let me briefly share my donors' stories:

- Sherrie – my wife, matched my blood type but was declined because she was considered pre-diabetic.

- Candace – Sherrie's sister, matched my blood type but was declined because she took a drug call Humera.

- Shanon – my daughter, not my blood type but was declined because she had kidney issues of her own (GFR <40).

- Sean – my son, not my blood type but was declined because he already took too many blood pressure medications.

- Hailey – my granddaughter, not my blood type and did not want to go into the Kidney Paired Exchange Program.

- Vicki – friend, not my blood type and did not want to participate in the Kidney Paired Exchange Program.

- Julie – friend, not my blood type and did not want to participate in the Kidney Paired Exchange Program.

- Brittany – friend, failed the online portion.

- Margie – friend (high school sweetheart), matched my blood type but decided she just couldn't go through with it.

- Robert – high school friend (and a doctor himself), matching blood type but was declined because of a heart procedure that involved a stent in his heart.

- Jacob – grandson, not a matching blood type and did not want to participate in the Kidney Paired Exchange Program.

- Tasha – cousin, matching blood type, but decided she just couldn't go through with it.

- Gillian – niece, matching blood type but took the remote tests and had a scare with her mammogram results, deciding not to proceed.

- Jennifer – my stepdaughter, not a matching blood type, but willing to move forward with the Kidney Paired Exchange Program.

- Lisa – a friend of Jennifer's, not my blood type, dropped out due to Covid.

- Bob Bevis – Sean's neighbor, failed the online test.

So, I had sixteen people offer me a kidney. How blessed am I? In the end, I had only one donor, Jennifer, who did not match my blood type but was willing to move forward on a Kidney Paired Exchange basis. To those donors who opted out I totally understand, and I hold no resentment towards them because of their decision. I'm not sure I would have been a donor if I were in their shoes. I love you for even considering giving me one of your kidneys.

My own son, Sean, who was not my blood type, but was disqualified for blood pressure medications, said he would not have participated in the Kidney Paired Exchange Program if he were eligible. He said, "Dad, if I can't give my kidney directly to you, then I don't think I want to give it to someone else." I get that. I understand that decision.

From January 2020 through May 2020, I was being tested by Emory doctors while my donors were at various stages of their own process. It was very stressful. I am not a patient person by nature, and it was very frustrating that the pace was so slow. I always thought I should go to the top of every list and always receive the highest priority. Don't these people know I have kidney disease?

The donor phase was equally stressful. Emory provides no feedback to recipients about their donors, not how many, not where they are in the testing, nothing! (Those HIPPA laws were protecting me from knowing anything about my donors.) The only feedback I received was from the donors directly.

With sixteen people, my hopes were high that one would be a match. Each week I learned that another candidate had been rejected, and I began to lose hope. Then when some were cleared to move forward but they opted out on their own, it always seemed like a devastating setback. However, I trusted God to provide a kidney.

During this time, I did not consider dialysis a viable alternative for me. I had all my eggs in the transplant basket. As donors were eliminated, my hopes for a new kidney diminished every week. Keeping a positive outlook was a challenge, yet I knew that God was in control. I had told God that all my trust was in Him. Psalm 9:10 says, "Those who know your name trust in you, for you, Lord, have never forsaken those who seek you."

While I would see doctors and get procedures done, my hope and trust were in the Lord, not in them. The same was true for my finances—my hope was in God, not my 401K.

"Those who trust in the Lord are like Mt. Zion, which cannot be shaken but endures forever" (Ps. 125:1).

The window of time from January 2020 to May 2020 was a season of great turmoil, full of agonizingly slow testing, donor feedback that seemed to sap my hope, trying to stay positive for my family, and constantly acknowledging my trust in God all along the way. Little did I know that my biggest disappointment was right around the corner!

Takeaways

1. *Your transplant coordinator needs to be your friend.* Reach out to them and make them see you as a person, not as a case number. Befriend them, learn their children's names, their hobbies, etc.

2. *Your donors must also go through a testing protocol* to be cleared to donate. Not everyone is eligible, so don't be disheartened when donors are eliminated. Be thankful they loved you enough to offer you one of their kidneys.

3. *Be sure your donors know about the Kidney Paired Exchange Program.* They don't have to be your blood type to participate. It expands your donor pool with a willing donor. However, some people just can't do this. My own son didn't want to do it, so don't be discouraged when some donors opt out of it.

4. *Be patient.* God taught me a lot about patience during this time.

5. *Don't neglect your family.* Let them support you, encourage you, and cry with you. Keep them informed and always up-to-date on where things stand. If they know, they can help. If they don't know, they can't help.

4

Test Results

Sometime in mid-April I got a call from Denise, my transplant coordinator, and she said that the MRI had shown a mass on one of my kidneys. They wanted me to see a urologist for a further opinion on it. They sent me to see a physician associate (PA) named Brenden Fels. I figured it must not be very bad if they sent me to a PA rather than an MD. Of course, it was another two weeks before I could get an appointment.

Brendon was a young guy and very tall, maybe 6'4" or more. He is very personable and I immediately liked him. The radiologist report from the MRI said that the mass presented and was consistent with renal cell carcinoma. Brenden confirmed that it was cancer.

I questioned him thoroughly. I asked, "What if the tumor is consistent with renal cell carcinoma, but not really renal cell carcinoma?"

After all, they had not done a biopsy, so they had no tissue or pathology report. He informed me that renal cell carcinoma has a distinct appearance on an MRI, and there was no doubt about the cancer.

Well, I freaked. I knew they didn't like to transplant patients with cancer, and I saw my hopes of a new kidney going down the drain.

My next question was, "What treatment plan do you recommend?" I knew Brendan would be sending a report to the transplant team about what he thought.

He said various options were available for treating renal cell carcinoma, including a nephrectomy (removal of the kidney) or a partial nephrectomy where only the part of the kidney with the carcinoma is removed.

Removing the entire kidney was out of the question for me. My GFR was already 16, and removal of a kidney would immediately take it to 8, and that would mean dialysis. The partial nephrectomy seemed like the only option to me.

I asked again, "What do you recommend?"

To my astonishment he said, "Nothing." He went on to say that the carcinoma was very small and very slow-growing. In situations like this, they recommend observation as the best treatment plan, with another MRI in a year to see if it had grown (more about that later).

Brendon's recommendation to the transplant team was to proceed with the kidney transplant and do another MRI in a year. The transplant team accepted his recommendation but with one caveat. Six weeks after the transplant, they wanted the kidney with the carcinoma to be totally removed. Because any transplant requires the patient to be on immunosuppressant drugs, any existing cancers can quickly get worse because the body has little or no immune system. I was okay with that, not that I had any choice.

I should note here that when one receives a kidney transplant, they do not replace an old kidney, nor do they put the new kidney in one's back near the old kidneys. They put the new kidney in one's lower abdomen in the front. They reroute blood flow and create a new connection to the bladder. It's an incredibly ingenious plan, and they have obviously perfected the procedure.

I was elated with this news, and my hopes for a new kidney were back on track. However, the second surgery to remove my old cancerous kidney concerned me. I hadn't really thought much about the transplant surgery, but now I did. It is not a simple surgery, there is the surgery itself, then a week to ten days in the hospital, then the immunosuppressant drugs, then many weeks of recovery. After that, I had to go back in and have my old kidney removed. And that surgery isn't necessarily easy either. These back-to-back major surgeries worried me. I was seventy-three years old, and that is a lot of anesthesia and trauma for someone my age! Nevertheless, it was full speed ahead! God seemed to be doing His thing and making a way forward.

Then Denise called me. She said the MRI also showed that my lymph nodes were enlarged. The transplant team wanted Dr. Friend to order a biopsy of my lymph nodes. Now remember, by this time, I'd already had a kidney biopsy and a bone marrow biopsy, and I wasn't thrilled about the idea of another biopsy. Neither was Dr. Friend.

Dr. Friend argued that the lymph nodes were only slightly enlarged and did not warrant a biopsy. The radiology department, who would have to do the biopsy under radiological guidance, agreed with Dr. Friend. Radiology also expressed concern that it was a difficult procedure at best. They would have to go in through my back, and it was a risky procedure for me. In fact, Dr. Friend had trouble finding a radiologist who would even perform the procedure, but eventually she found a radiologist willing to do it.

My confidence level was not very high given that my oncologist didn't think it was necessary, and the radiologist thought it was risky. Nonetheless, the transplant team wanted the biopsy to complete their work-up on me before deciding about whether to clear me for transplant.

The transplant team basically told Dr. Friend and radiology that unless my lymph nodes were biopsied, there would be no transplant.

Denise brought a new perspective from the transplant team that I hadn't considered before. I was a patient that had a renal cell carcinoma and an inconclusive bone marrow biopsy with a B-cell anomaly. They had to know if any other cancer was present. Their team was looking beyond the actual surgery to how I would do on immunosuppressant drugs. Plus, if it was cancer, how long had it been there and what was the stage of the cancer?

From the transplant team's perspective, additional pathology was needed when considering the lifelong impact of adding immunosuppression to the patient's medications and the management of that medication when cancer is part of the equation. While Dr. Friend may not need that information to treat the cancer, the transplant team needed it to make candidacy decisions. Oncologists may not always be happy about that.

This back and forth between Dr. Friend and the transplant team took another month before they actually did the biopsy. I remember meeting with Dr. Friend and I told her, "These transplant surgeons seem to be only focused on their numbers and the percentage of their successful surgeries." The reality, however, was that I was a patient of both, and they were both trying to do what was medically best for me from their perspective in their chosen specialty.

Finally, the lymph node biopsy was scheduled. I was under sedation and thankfully don't remember a thing. They went in through my back, and it was sore for a couple of days. About a week later I had a follow-up meeting with Dr. Friend to learn the results of the biopsy. Dr. Friend didn't beat around the bush and told me straight-up that the pathology showed I had B-cell non-Hodgkin Lymphoma. My heart sank!

She drew me a few pictures that showed me how my lymphoma was considered "marginal zone," which is the lowest grade. However, the danger was that it could move to more severe levels at any time. I don't know if the transplant team ever said, "See, I told you so" to Dr. Friend. In any case, we were all glad that we had done the biopsy, but I was devastated about having another cancer.

I asked Dr. Friend what the treatment plan was for marginal zone B-cell non-Hodgkin Lymphoma. She said, "Nothing! In these cases we just observe the patient and when they become symptomatic, we begin the appropriate treatment." I was delighted to hear this, but I had serious doubts about whether the transplant team was going to move forward with a transplant on someone who now had two types of cancer.

This tested my faith. Back at home, I questioned God about what was going on. That's when I had my Jehoshaphat moment! Jehoshaphat was the King of Judah, and his story is found in 2 Chronicles 20. Jehoshaphat was surrounded by three armies, all ready to attack. He turned to God and said, "There is danger all around us. We are powerless against these vast armies. And we don't know what to do. But our eyes are on you" (v. 12). God then answered Jehoshaphat through a prophet who said, "Do not be afraid or discouraged because of this vast army. For the battle is not yours, but God's" (v. 15).

And I felt just like Jehoshaphat. I was not surrounded by three armies but by renal cell carcinoma, B-Cell non-Hodgkin

Lymphoma, and end-stage renal failure. My hopes of a new kidney seemed to be disappearing quickly. I told God I was scared and didn't know what to do. Then I realized that Jehoshaphat's answer was my answer. This was God's battle. What am I going to do against cancer and renal failure? I felt sudden peace. It was if God said, "Steve, don't worry another minute about your health. I've got this! I've heard your prayers and thousands of others praying on your behalf. Don't worry, I've got this. I want you to write another book." Because I believe He does have it, I wrote another book (more on the book later).

Treatment Plan

Dr. Friend then wrote to the transplant team about her treatment plan for my lymphoma. She recommended they move forward with the transplant. (This may have partially been due to the fact that she knew I was very opposed to dialysis.) But the transplant team did not buy in to her recommendation. Her argument was to do the transplant and if the lymphoma got worse, she would treat it, but at least I would have a new kidney to help me fight the cancer.

The Book

About this same time I got a call from Joyce Hill, a young woman I graduated from high school with in 1965. She found me on Facebook and saw that I was a Jesus follower and an author. She asked me where she could get my books, and I told her they were available on Amazon. She bought both books, read them, and called me back to tell me that she really enjoyed them. She asked if I had any ideas for future books.

I told her I did have some ideas. My first book was a book on psychology and how we all see the world through a lens. Each person's lens is different, and on our lens, we place all the things that we hold to be true. During my life I had observed many things that people believed about religion (God, church, the Bible, etc.) that I didn't think were true. I wanted to write a book about those things and why I believed they weren't true.

I shared this idea with Joyce and she liked it. I learned that Joyce was a journalism major in college and had worked at several jobs where her duties required editing. It just seemed too much of a coincidence to me, so I asked her if would be interested in coauthoring the book with me. She accepted. In addition to all my doctor appointments, for the next several months I was writing another book.

Conference

The transplant coordinator meets weekly with the transplant team in what they call a "conference" or sometimes "committee." At the conference, the coordinator updates the team on how the patient is progressing through all the testing and meeting with medical personal and other staff. Usually they meet weekly, and Denise would give me an update on next steps. But things really slowed down with Dr. Friend's recommendation.

The transplant team and Dr. Friend went back and forth for a long time, nearly a month. I had no visibility into their debate. Denise was unable to provide any feedback during this time. It was agonizing to wait for an answer.

The transplant surgeon and transplant nephrologist (a different nephrologist from Dr. Gowda) will often go against a specialists' recommendation if they believe the chances of a poor outcome are likely. The question they always ask themselves is, "Do the risks of transplant outweigh the benefits?" It is not just about the surgery itself. If they believe the patient will do poorly on immunosuppressant drugs, then they will oftentimes decline the surgery.

Denise says there are many cases where a patient regrets getting a transplant because they develop some post-op complication like infection or cancer, and they wish they hadn't done the transplant. After a transplant, a person can always go back on dialysis, but you can't go back and get off the immunosuppressant drugs.

Even when a transplanted kidney fails, the recipient may remain on low doses of immunosuppression to keep them from building up antibodies to that kidney. Developing antibodies makes finding a match very difficult the second or third time around. Once a person has a transplanted kidney, no matter what new health issues may come up during their life, immunosuppression will have to play a part in that treatment.

Regardless of what the transplant team decided, at least I knew that God had it. Finally, Denise called me and told me the transplant team had made a final decision. I was on pins and needles.

Takeaways

1. *If they find something wrong in your testing (and send you to other specialists for further opinion) don't assume the worst*, as I did. Many times these conditions are treatable and won't impact your transplant.

5

The Final Word

Dr. Friend was going to have to argue long and hard if she were going to change the transplant team's mind. And God bless her, she did. I don't know whether it was her persistence where she just became the squeaky wheel that got oiled, or whether her medical arguments and my opposition to dialysis carried the day, but she won!

The Emory transplant team cleared me to receive a new kidney. Whatever argument Dr. Friend made, it was compelling enough for the transplant team to approve me. I couldn't believe it. My PCP couldn't believe it, and Dr. Gowda couldn't believe it. The National Kidney Foundation and Emory put me the waitlist for a new kidney.

Dr. Friend was elated about me getting cleared for transplant. I knew she had worked hard on my behalf and I was very appreciative. As it now relates to my lymphoma, Dr. Friend is really waiting for me to become symptomatic before beginning any treatment. The typical symptoms I might display are weight loss, fever, chills, night sweats, lymph node growth or pain, or blood work where my hemoglobin drops below 10. The difficulty with these symptoms is that they are easily attributable to other causes, especially Covid.

This news was everything I had been praying for, and thousands of others had been praying for as well. James 5:16 says,

Therefore confess your sins to each other and pray for each other that you may be healed. The prayer of a righteous person is powerful and effective.

I clearly had some righteous people praying for me.

I should note here that all my other doctors were very shocked to learn that I was cleared for transplant with two cancers. Dr. Gowda said she was very surprised and so was my PCP, Dr. Phil Rogers.

At this point, my focus totally shifted to my donor pool. Nothing was more important for me to do now that I had been cleared and approved for a transplant. As I noted earlier, in Georgia the wait time for a deceased donor is about seven years, so I was really hoping that one of my donors could get cleared, and we could get the surgery scheduled as quickly as possible.

I asked Denise how common it was for a patient with two cancers to get cleared for a kidney transplant. She said, "It is not rare, but the key is the type of cancer, the pathology, the stage, and the treatment they are receiving. It used to be an automatic rejection because of fear the cancer would spread once on immunotherapy. But today it is fairly common to consider patients for transplant with a history of cancer."

And then, Emory suddenly stopped all non-emergency surgeries, including transplants, because of COVID-19. My donors were encouraged to continue their testing protocols in hopes that surgeries would resume in a short time. This was a terrific mental and emotional blow to me, with no apparent end in sight. No one knew how long Covid would affect the surgical schedule. I prayed that God would give me patience, and please give it to me right now! Again, I was reminded of Romans 8:25: "But if we hope for what we do not yet have, we wait for it patiently."

In June of 2020, about half my donors had been eliminated for one reason or another. By August I was down to just two—my stepdaughter Jennifer and her friend, Lisa (who to this day I have never met). Lisa, who was not my blood type anyway, was spooked by Covid, and Emory wasn't doing transplants anyway. Lisa just went into a holding pattern and Jennifer, bless her heart, decided to move forward on a Kidney Paired Exchange basis.

About this time I had a follow-up meeting with Dr. Friend. She wanted to do another PET scan. The results did not show the lymphoma since I was in the marginal zone, but we knew I had it because we had the tissue and the pathology.

By now, I knew that Dr. Friend was responsible for me being cleared for a transplant, which of course meant that I would be going on the immunosuppressant drugs after surgery. I asked Dr. Friend, "What are the chances that my cancers will 'blossom' once I'm on the immunosuppressant drugs?" (The word blossom is her term, not mine, and it means it will spread and get worse.)

Her immediate answer was, "Nothing is one-hundred percent, but it is very high." I practically fell off my chair.

"Very high?" I asked in disbelief.

She said, "Yes. People with no cancer at all, who go on immunosuppressant drugs, are five times more likely to get cancer than those not on immunosuppressant drugs. They have no immune system to fight with. We can treat your cancer with chemo and other drugs, but I can almost promise you we will be treating you because your cancer will very likely blossom."

Well, you could have knocked me over with a feather. First of all, I wasn't looking forward to transplant surgery in the first place, then the drugs and the recovery. Second, I was going to have to have a second surgery to remove my kidney with the renal cell carcinoma. And now third, I was going to be treated for worsening cancer. As much as I hated the thought of dialysis, it seemed to be looking like a more reasonable alternative after all.

I asked Dr. Friend, "If I were your father (and I could easily be, based on age), what would you advise your dad to do—transplant or dialysis?" She thought for a moment and said, "I'd advise him against a transplant. I would tell him to work with his nephrologist to make his kidneys last as long as possible, and then go on dialysis. You can live a long productive life on dialysis." She said this knowing that I was not a big proponent of dialysis. I think she was being totally transparent and truthful.

I thanked Dr. Friend for her honesty and went home to share all that I had just learned with Sherrie. We discussed it for several days. We talked through all the pros and cons of each approach, the donor situation, plus the option to make no decision at that time. In the whole journey and saga of my kidney disease this was, without doubt, the second biggest decision I had to make.

The biggest argument for a transplant was the freedom I would have after the surgery to live a relatively normal life. I would have to take immunosuppressant drugs every day, but that was certainly not a burdensome responsibility. I valued Dr. Friend's advice, though. This is a doctor who treats cancer for a living, and I could see her telling her dad, "Dad, I do this for living. While I can treat cancer, I don't invite it. Your lymphoma is marginal zone and could stay that way forever. Let's just make your kidneys last as long as possible and then do dialysis. You can live a long and full life as a dialysis patient."

On the other hand, I could also see her saying, "Dad, I do this for living. Get the transplant, and I'll personally treat your cancer. We can do this."

Another big component of the decision was my donor situation. I loved the relatives that came forward to offer me a kidney. They're really saying, "I love you enough to give you one of my kidneys. I want to save your life." What incredible generosity! At the same time, transplant is a very serious surgery. The donor is in the hospital several days, with another week or so before they can return to driving or go back to work.

In my case, my last and only donor, who was not my blood type, was my stepdaughter Jennifer. If something happened to her during surgery, what would I say to Sherrie? Was Sherrie even willing to let Jennifer go through with it? What about Jennifer's husband, Scott? How could I ever look him in the eye again if something happened to her? Was he even willing to let her do it? I was also uneasy about my two grandsons, Karsten and Trevor. If something happened, how could I tell them that their mom died while saving my life? They'd definitely rather have her back than me! I just wasn't sure I could even ask her to go through with it.

I was also concerned about my age. The idea of giving someone my age, with cancer, a new kidney didn't seem right to me. If I received a new kidney and lived for six months, only to then die from cancer, that seemed selfish to me. Forty-year-old moms are out there with kids and no cancer, who could probably live forty years on the same kidney. Again, it just didn't seem right.

These are agonizing decisions. Family and a lot of love are involved. What is the right thing to do? I asked God to give me guidance, and Psalm 25 was my guide.

Show me your ways, Lord, teach me your paths. Guide me in your truth and teach me, for you are God my Savior, and my hope is in you all day long (vv. 4-5).

When all was said and done, and considering all the tangential issues, I decided that dialysis was the right decision for me and my family. All my concern about Jennifer as a donor went away. My choice lined up with Dr. Friend's advice, and I valued her opinion. Even though she argued hard (and won) and got me cleared for a transplant, I think it was because she knew I hated the thought of dialysis.

I really didn't want a second surgery to remove a kidney with the renal cell carcinoma or the inevitable fight with cancer. I just needed to come to grips with being kept alive by a machine. When I told Sherrie what I decided, she said she thought I made a very wise decision.

All I had to do now was tell everyone else!

Takeaways

1. *If you get cleared for a transplant, congratulations!* Start working immediately with your donors. Due to HIPPA laws, the transplant coordinator and the donor coordinator cannot share any information with you about donors. All your feedback must come from the donor. Let your donors know this, and ask them to please keep you informed about where they are in the testing process.

2. *Delays are inevitable.* Count on it. In my case, the big delay was Covid. Don't be discouraged. Remain patient and eventually things will begin to move forward again.

3. *With your doctors, make a reasonable judgment about how your life will be once you are on immunosuppressant drugs.* For me,

my cancer posed a post-op risk, and needing chemo was a consideration. Discuss the pros/cons with your family and others whose wisdom you value. Be honest.

4. *It's okay to opt out of transplant* if your expected post-op life on immunosuppressant drugs is questionable. It's a risk with either choice (transplant vs. dialysis). You just have to be honest with yourself about the pros and cons of each option and choose the one best for you.

5. This was one of my toughest decisions. *Seek God's guidance.* Perhaps God wants you to write a book!

6

Expert Advice about Transplants

I met with Denise Neal, my transplant coordinator, for over three hours on a Sunday afternoon. What follows is some of the expert advice she shared with me.

If you are eligible for a kidney transplant and thinking about entering the testing protocol to get cleared and placed on the waiting list, the most important thing you need to do is become educated about transplants.

What most patients miss is a complete understanding of the post-operative world of a transplant recipient. The top risks include rejection of the organ, infection, and the risks of cancer while on immunosuppression drugs. Some patients who get a transplant find that they are sicker than when they were on dialysis. The biggest tragedy is when a patient wishes they had never stopped dialysis. You can go back on dialysis, but immunosuppressant drugs are forever, and you can't go back and change it.

Try to find a living donor so the transplant can happen early in your diagnosis. The best option is to secure a transplant before you go on dialysis. Family donors are welcome and have a higher chance of a matching blood type, but tradeoffs are involved, just as I had with Jennifer. Just because a family member matches your blood type, it doesn't mean that person is an eligible donor. A cross-match test is required, and a negative result means the kidney is compatible.

The transplant team is always looking at the likely post-op experience. For me, a guy with two cancers, my projected post-op experience was that I would likely have to have chemo treatments because of the immunosuppressant drugs. The doctors maximize the immunosuppressant drug dosage at the beginning and then begin a tapering process. By regularly checking blood work, they can tell when your creatinine levels begin to increase. At that point, they stop the taper, and that dosage becomes your dosage for life.

Sometimes this taper process can take six months. If cancer develops in those six months and chemo treatments begin, the transplant team is always worried about the effect of the chemo on the new kidney.

The transplant team is always asking the question, "Is the risk of the transplant greater than the benefit?" In my case, the answer was yes.

Patients should be realistic about the recurrence of their original disease. In my case, the recurrence of cancer was highly likely, and I had to be realistic about that.

Transplant patients need to understand the importance of their role in a successful transplant. They must be committed to following directions, taking their meds faithfully, and taking full ownership of their own healthcare. Taking a break from the post-op regimen can mean losing the transplanted kidney.

Patients also need to understand that they are not getting a new kidney. That kidney had a previous owner and a history that you may know nothing about. Many deceased donor organs have a history that cannot be known. When information is available, you may learn that the donor was a drug addict or had some other high-risk condition or lifestyle. I signed a form that said I would consider a high risk donor, mainly because I had sixteen living donors, and I didn't think I would ever need a deceased donor kidney.

Finally, never forget and never fail to appreciate what your donor is gifting to you. It says a lot about what someone thinks of you to offer you one of their organs. It says, "I'm willing to give you a part of me in order to save your life." If you are receiving a deceased donor kidney, remember a family is grieving a family member somewhere, and I would pray for them.

Takeaways

1. *Listen to all the expert advice before making your decisions.* Understand all the risks and possible consequences. Seek God's counsel. Here is Paul's advice from Philippians 4:6,

   Do not be anxious about anything, but in every situation, by prayer and petition, with thanksgiving, present your requests to God. And the peace of God, which transcends all understanding, will guard your hearts and your minds in Christ Jesus.

7

Coming to Grips with Dialysis

After Sherrie, the first person I told about deciding to not have a transplant was my only remaining donor, Jennifer. I think she was relieved, and I'm sure Sherrie and Scott were also. I'm not sure how much my two grandsons knew about the transplant and/or Jennifer's potential role. My guess is that they knew very little at that time because surgery in the Kidney Paired Exchange Program was at least six months away anyhow.

The next person I told was Dr. Friend. She had argued so effectively on my behalf and was really responsible for me getting cleared for transplant in the first place. I was worried that she would be angry with me because of all her efforts to get me approved. She understood, though, and was glad I was opting for dialysis. She supported my decision, but I know it broke her heart. In some ways I feel like I let her down, but in the end, it was the right decision for me.

The next person I told was my nephrologist, Dr. Gowda. She was also supportive of my decision. She again expressed her surprise that the transplant team had even cleared me with two cancers. I also told my PCP, Dr. Phil Rogers. He too again expressed his surprise that the transplant team had cleared me, and he also supported my decision.

Finally, I told Denise to take me off the wait list. I asked her for her thoughts about my decision.

She said, "I was sorry to hear that you were not going to be transplanted. You had been through so much testing and waiting. But I never want a patient to go through all that and then have a bad outcome. Once a transplant is done, it is done. There is no going back. You would be on immunosuppressant drugs for the rest of your life. The finality of it can make living with rejection, infection, or cancer a nightmare. I think you made an informed decision, and I'm relieved by your choice."

Denise went on to say, "The most challenging cases are those that include medical comorbidities, social issues, or financial issues. These patients are sick and overwhelmed. They just don't have the wherewithal to get everything done in a timely manner. Not everyone has family and social support to assist them, and this is probably the saddest thing to see.

"Most often the people who remove themselves from the transplant list are older and realize that dialysis three times a week will be easier than the complicated post-operative requirements that come with a transplant."

About this time in September 2020, Dr. Friend ordered another PET scan. It showed that my lymphoma was still considered marginal zone. My hope was that it would stay that way for a long time. In fact, it's possible that I've had B-cell non-Hodgkin lymphoma for thirty plus years and just never knew it. The same is true for the renal cell carcinoma. I was just thankful that the treatment plan for the time being was just observation.

I met again with Dr. Gowda to learn more about my dialysis options. She set me up for a class at the Pure Life Renal Dialysis Clinic. Sherrie and I went together, and the class was conducted by Nurse Tonya Rolle. She did a great job of explaining my options, and Sherrie and I left with a lot of literature to read. I had no idea how many options I really had, and all the options required surgery before dialysis could even begin.

The two basic options are hemodialysis and peritoneal dialysis. With hemodialysis, you go to a dialysis clinic three times per week for approximately four hours. However, prior to starting hemodialysis, you need a shunt in your arm. This shunt can be either a fistula or an AV graft, which serves as the necessary access point for dialysis treatments.

The fistula combines one's own vein and artery. This creates a larger passageway that allows for increased blood flow, thus allowing more blood to be cleansed at each dialysis treatment. In contrast, the AV graft uses an artificial tubing to connect the vein and artery. Usually, the fistula takes six to eight weeks to fully mature before it can be used.

Peritoneal dialysis can be done at home. It also requires surgery to insert a catheter in your peritoneal cavity prior to starting dialysis. The advantages to peritoneal dialysis are the flexibility to do it at home, and to do it at night while you sleep. Usually, it is done seven days per week for nine hours each day.

Another benefit is that you can travel more easily. The negatives seem to be proneness for greater risk of infection, the possible need for assistance (depending on your condition), the complexity and size of the machine, and carrying a twenty-pound machine with you wherever you travel. Plus, you must have a large storage area for the supplies that are needed, as every month you receive thirty boxes of supplies, which are heavy and 1 foot x 2 feet x 1 foot in dimension.

You should go online and read all you can about these two fundamental alternatives. A great deal of technical information is available, and now you can even do hemodialysis at home, if you are comfortable with inserting your own needles.

In the end, I chose hemodialysis. My fundamental reasoning was I didn't want to have to do anything, know anything, or learn anything. I just wanted to show up somewhere, let them stick me, wait for four hours, and then go home. It just seemed like the easiest way to start. At a later date, I may change my mind and switch to peritoneal but not anytime soon. When I told Dr. Gowda of my choice, she seemed a little surprised. I guess for whatever reason, she thought I would prefer peritoneal.

Dr. Gowda said she thought I was a good candidate for peritoneal dialysis because my condition would allow me to do it. Not everyone is physically or mentally able to do peritoneal dialysis, but it is an option for many people.

I told Dr. Gowda that I would like to move forward with the vascular surgery to create the fistula that would serve as my access for dialysis treatments. Since it takes six to eight weeks for the fistula to mature, and since we didn't really know how long my kidneys would last on their own, I was anxious to do it sooner rather than later to avoid any emergency. Dr. Gowda agreed completely. This turned out to be one of the best decisions we made.

Dr. Gowda set me up for an appointment with a vascular surgeon named Dr. Peter H'doubler. The first thing he did was a procedure that they call "vein mapping." It's an ultrasound scan with a handheld wand that measures the size and location of the veins and arteries. It also measures the thickness of the vein/artery walls and their depth from the surface of the skin. They begin with your non-dominant arm, which for me was my left arm since I'm right-handed.

If the veins/arteries weren't suitable, they would have moved to my right arm. Fortunately for me, my left arm had great veins and arteries. I met with Dr. H'doubler, who walked me through what the procedure would be, how long it would take, and the results he was hoping to achieve. We scheduled the surgery for about two weeks out, and the surgery was done on September 21, 2020.

Dialysis Treatments

During dialysis, nurses insert two needles in your arm, and the needles are attached to individual tubing, which in turn are attached to the dialysis machine. Once the needles are inserted, blood leaves the body through one tubing, gets cleaned by the dialysis machine, and the cleansed blood reenters the body through the second tubing.

Missing Dialysis Treatments

On average, a dialysis patient dialyzes three times a week for an average of four hours per treatment (twelve hours per week). The treatment replaces the work that your kidneys perform on a twenty-four/seven basis (168 hours per week). Dialysis is trying to do in twelve hours what your kidneys do in 168 hours. Therefore, missing minutes of dialysis decreases the results and increases the likelihood of complications and hospitalizations.

Your dialysis treatments replace only a small amount of the work your kidneys do to remove fluid and waste products. If you don't get enough dialysis, your blood accumulates that fluid and waste. Over time, waste and fluid can build up to a lethal amount.

When you miss dialysis:
- You may feel weak, tired, and have shortness of breath while moving around.

- You can develop a metallic taste in your mouth.
- You lose your appetite and feel nauseated.
- You may develop swelling in your ankles, stomach, or other areas.
- You have a taste of ammonia in your mouth.
- You may have prolonged bleeding times after dialysis.

Additionally, if patients miss, or shorten, three or more dialysis treatments in a month, then you have:

- A higher risk of hospitalization.
- A risk of life-threatening complications.
- A greater risk of being removed from the transplant list.
- A greater risk of infection.
- Fluid accumulation around your heart, causing it to swell and risk further heart conditions.

The effects on your health from less dialysis may not show up overnight. You may not feel ill until you experience lasting health effects on your body. For example, you may not notice the extra fluid building up in your body, but it will make your heart pump harder, which can cause it to enlarge and possibly fail. Missing one treatment per month is the equivalent of missing a whole month of treatment over a year. Shortening your time by one hour each treatment is the equivalent of missing thirty-six treatments per year. It adds up quickly.

One of the things you need to know is that on dialysis you need to monitor your fluid intake. You are only allowed thirty-two ounces per day. Dialysis can only remove so much fluid per treatment (and you will cramp if too much fluid is removed). You don't want the fluid to build up in your body because that will cause other problems. Be aware that anything that melts at room temperature is considered a fluid, such as ice cream and JELL-O.

The patients who are successful at staying with the recommended treatment regimen usually have a good plan of how to maximize their time. They watch TV, play card games, read, or sleep if they have an early chair time. My chair time is 5:30–9:30 a.m., and I'm often able to sleep some of the time.

If you have an emergency, just work with the clinic staff to reschedule your treatment so you don't miss any dialysis time.

The Book

It was about this same time in late September a year after my vascular surgery that Joyce and I finished writing the book. I was looking for a publisher but quickly realized that publishers don't just accept manuscripts directly from authors. They only accept manuscripts from literary agents. The agents screen out all the junk, so the publisher knows the material is decent if an agent has agreed to represent the book. I started looking for a Christian agent, since this was going to be considered a religious book.

I talked with several agents, and I really liked this one guy in Pennsylvania named Keith Carroll. He is a retired pastor, had written several books, and now just helped new authors get published.

Keith said, "Send me the manuscript and one hundred dollars for my time to read it, and then we'll have a two-hour conference call in which I'll tell you everything I think about your book—the good, the bad, and the ugly."

It sounded like a deal.

About three weeks later, I received an email that he was ready to schedule our conference call. Joyce and I got on a three-way call and I said, "Well, Keith, what did you think of the book?"

His immediate reply was, "I hated it." I was shocked. The book was based on all the things I had heard people say about God, the Bible, faith, church, or anything else religious, that I thought was wrong and not really what the Bible taught. Keith said, "Who wants to read a book, let alone pay for it, that tells them why everything they believe is wrong and why everything you think is right?" I had to agree nobody would want to read a book like that.

Keith said that he thought we had some good material in the book, but the context was just not good. He said if we were willing to rewrite the book from a different perspective, he would read the new version at no cost, and we'd have another conference call after he read it. It seemed very fair.

I was devastated by Keith's reaction, and my ego was really bruised. I couldn't even discuss it with Joyce. I had to digest it myself first. I went to sleep praying, "God, you told me to write a book and I did; you brought me a coauthor; you found us a literary agent, and he hates it. What's going on, Lord?" About 5:30 a.m. in the morning, in the twilight area between sleep and consciousness, I heard God whisper to me, "Steve, just tell them about Me."

I sat straight up in bed. I immediately knew the title of the book—*The God I Know*. I was going to tell people everything I knew about God—His attitude, attributes, personality, what brings Him joy, how He acts in certain situations, and everything I knew about Him. I went to my computer and in thirty minutes wrote the introduction.

You see, Christianity is not about religion, it is about relationship. God wants a relationship with His children. But you can't have a relationship with someone you don't know. If I could tell people about the God I know, then maybe they might want a relationship with Him too. So I told Joyce what God had given me and that I wanted to rewrite the book. She totally agreed when I told her how it all happened.

In September and October of 2020, Joyce and I rewrote the book. We sent it back to Keith and he loved it. He suggested we add a subtitle of, "And the Relationship We Need," which was perfect. He said he would put a ribbon around it and send it off to some publishers. In late November, I received an email from Keith that River Birch Press in Alabama wanted to publish the book, and that I would be a receiving a contract offer from Brian Banashak, the publisher.

I was just over the moon to actually have a publisher for our book, and Joyce was about to become a published author.

Brian told me he could have the book in my hands by March 1, 2021. This gave us time to build a website, find a fulfillment house, and create a sales, marketing, and promotional plan.

All was good. The book was being published, my kidneys were functioning at about 15%, and it looked like my kidneys would last perhaps another year before I would need dialysis. The holidays were approaching, and everything seemed to be looking good.

Little did I know the devastation that January 1, 2021, would bring, which was right around the corner.

Takeaways

1. *Neither transplant nor dialysis is a bad decision.* Each situation is different, and so many factors are part of the decision. Talk with your family and choose the option that is best for you.

2. *Read all you can about the various types of dialysis,* and the pros and cons of each option. Hemodialysis involves needles and is usually done three times per week for four hours. Peritoneal dialysis uses no needles but must be done every day for nine hours—but you can do it at night while you sleep. Go to Amia.com and watch a fifteen-minute video on the peritoneal process. Pick the dialysis treatment that is best for you.

3. *Both hemodialysis and peritoneal require surgery.* For hemodialysis you need vascular surgery to create what they call a fistula, which is your access and where to place the needles. Peritoneal dialysis requires abdominal surgery where a port is created for daily treatment.

4. *If you choose hemodialysis, move forward with the vascular surgery quickly.* You never know when your kidneys will fail. Mine failed earlier than I thought. I believed I had another year before I would need dialysis, but because I had a mature fistula, I was able to start dialysis in the hospital in a non-emergency situation.

5. *Don't skip dialysis treatments.* They are not always convenient and sometimes you will want to skip them, but don't do it. They are essential for your overall health.

6. *Find things to do during your kidney ordeal.* I wrote a book, but you could do anything. Keep busy and occupy your life with life—not kidney disease. This helps relieve the stress and worry about your medical condition.

7. *Now is a good time to get to know God better,* develop and deepen your faith, and put all your trust and hope in Him.

8

Fighting for My Life

On January 1, 2021, I contracted COVID-19. We had a few people over that day to watch college football, including my daughter, Jennifer, her husband, Scott, and their twin boys, Karsten and Trevor. My former business partner, Steve Bacastow, and his wife, Kim, also joined us. We all felt fine. Georgia beat Cincinnati 24-21, and everybody eventually went home. By the next day, I started feeling ill. All of us there that day eventually were stricken with COVID-19. We have no idea where or who exposed us all to the virus.

My case was by far the worst. By January 3rd, Sherrie had to call the EMTs to come take me to the hospital. I was not very responsive to verbal commands, I couldn't walk, and Sherrie could not get me in the car. She had called Jen and Scott to come help her, but before they arrived, she called the EMTs. Much of that time is hazy to me, but I remember being loaded into the back of the ambulance when Scott and Jen drove up. I gave them a wave, but it was all I could do. Jennifer told Sherrie later that I looked so bad she didn't think she would ever see me alive again.

In the emergency room I was unresponsive. I lost all control of my bladder and bowels. I was having trouble breathing, I was running a fever, and I had no taste or smell. They put me on a heart monitor and discovered that I had gone into Atrial

Fibrillation (Afib). They started me on Eliquis® (a blood thinner) because Afib is known to throw blood clots. My oxygen level was in the low 80s, so the nurse started me on oxygen. My nose was clogged and bleeding. Finally, after five hours in the emergency room, I was moved into a room on a COVID-19 floor.

Since I was becoming dehydrated, I was started on an IV. Later that night, I felt well enough to call Sherrie and tell her my room number. It wasn't more than a five-minute call. The next morning doctors began descending on me: cardiologists, nephrologists, internists, and psychologists. I had no idea what they were doing, and I was too weak to care. I wasn't getting any better.

I prayed earnestly for healing and very specifically for the symptoms I was suffering from with Covid. A story in Luke 18 describes a blind man who was begging Jesus to have mercy on him. A large crowd surrounded Jesus, and He ordered the people to bring the blind man to Him. Jesus asked the blind man, "What do you want me to do for you?" The man quickly replied, "Lord, I want to see" (vv. 40-41). The prayer was short, specific, and to the point.

That is the way I like to pray, and I encourage you to do the same. Tell God specifically what you want or need. Jesus replied to the man, "Receive your sight; your faith has healed you" (v. 42). The blind man immediately received his sight and followed Jesus, praising God. When all the people saw it, they also praised God (v. 43).

After a week in the hospital, I really needed a shower. I hadn't bathed, shaved, or brushed my teeth in a week, and for the most part didn't care. I told the nurse I wanted to take a shower. She said that was not possible because I was unable to do it. I was also wearing a heart monitor, and those wires would have to be removed. The shower in my room had a seat in it, and I told her I was getting a shower with or without her help. She wasn't happy, but she went and put on her rubber hazmat suit. I guess she thought she was going to have to get in the shower with me.

The nurse helped me use my walker to get into the bathroom, and with the seat down, I sat on the toilet. I was then able to hold a handrail and move over to sit on the shower seat. Then I closed the shower curtain, took off my pajamas, and turned on the water. It felt so good. I washed my hair and body and just let the warm water run over me for about ten minutes. Then my nurse handed me a towel and some clean pajamas, and I made it back to my sink using my walker and shaved and brushed my teeth. When I got back into bed, I was exhausted. I thanked the nurse for her help and said, "See, I told you we could do it."

While in the hospital, breathing remained difficult, and I was only able to get an hour of sleep at night. I had no appetite. I literally ate nothing for days. From New Year's Day to Valentine's Day (forty-five days), I lost thirty-eight pounds. I had trouble standing, and I was very unstable on my feet. I could not get to the bathroom, so I was using a urinal all the time. I wore a wristband that said I was a "fall risk." I could not use my walker without help, and I wasn't allowed to move from my bed to an adjacent chair without help. I was in deep tapioca!

All this time, while I was in the hospital, Sherrie was at home getting worse and worse. Jennifer and Vicki Willard, a close and dear friend, were taking care of her. They finally took Sherrie to the hospital, and they admitted her too. She was discharged five days later but still needed a lot of care. Without Jen and Vicki, I don't know what we'd have done.

I called Joyce and basically turned the whole book project over to her. I told her I was down for the count and probably would not be able to work on it for several months.

I also have to say that I was not a very good patient. I am ashamed to say it, but I was not very kind to the nurses who were trying to take care of me. The main reason was that I was angry—at everything! I was angry that I was sick, angry that I couldn't see my family, angry that I had cancer and end-stage renal failure. I was just short-tempered and mad that I was in the hospital.

Then I heard the worst news. My kidneys had failed, and Dr. Gowda wanted me to start on dialysis right away in the hospital. I was in total agreement. I believed that Covid was killing me and that any help for my kidneys might just make me feel a little better. Because of my Covid, I was not allowed in the dialysis area, so they brought a dialysis machine to my room.

Needing dialysis so urgently, our decision to do the vascular surgery earlier made us look very smart. While at the time it seemed like an emergency dialysis, in Dr. Friend's mind it was inevitable that one day I would need dialysis anyway. She did not see my dialysis as a temporary remedy to help me get over Covid but as a repeated treatment for the rest of my life. She believes that Covid definitely hastened my kidney function decline.

My first dialysis was the worst experience of my life. First, I didn't really know what to expect. The nurse performing the dialysis was a female and looked to be no more than twenty-five years old. I wondered if I were her first patient! Putting the needles in was some of the worst pain I have ever experienced. They use a fourteen-gauge needle that is about the size of a fire hose. My brother said they use smaller needles on horses.

I'm sure my pain was compounded by the fact I had Covid and was flat on my back in a hospital bed. (The dialysis clinics all have reclining chairs with armrests.) Two days later they tried again, and the experience was even worse. I was only being dialyzed for two or three hours, but it was so awful it seemed like two weeks.

Two days later, they tried to perform a third treatment. This time they took me to the hospital's dialysis unit, but they put me in an isolation unit for the treatment. It was another young female. She got the first needle in okay, but she couldn't get the second needle into my arm. She said she thought my vein had collapsed. A fistula is a very large vein/artery combined.

Well, I lost it! I told her that Ray Charles could see that vein. I told her to take out the first needle and take me back to my room. I confess that I was rude and belligerent. This dialysis thing was a joke. She brought doctors in to try and change my mind, but I was done.

I am ashamed of my attitude and my actions, which were certainly not a Christian response to my situation. I trusted in God, but I took my eyes off Him and started focusing on my situation. I was angry about having cancer and kidney disease; I was angry that I had Covid and was in the hospital; I was angry that I felt so miserable; and I was angry that I couldn't see my family. When I realized I'd lost focus, I returned my eyes to my Lord, and my attitude changed.

When I arrived back in my room, I told the nurse that I wanted to speak to the doctor on duty. It was a Sunday. About thirty minutes later, he walked into my room.

I said, "Please prepare my discharge papers, I'm going home. Call my social worker and have them contact home hospice and have them meet me at my house."

He tried to talk me out of leaving, but I was having none of it. I told him, "I've been in here for a month and I'm no better. In fact, I may be worse. I can't stand dialysis; therefore, I'm going to die, and I'm not going to die alone in this hospital where I can't see my wife and family."

He said, "Obviously we can't keep you against your wishes; but if you leave, you will have to sign a form that says you are leaving against medical advice."

I said, "Fine, bring me the paperwork."

Sherrie was still sick with Covid, so she couldn't come get me. That duty fell to Jennifer. She was given permission to come to my room in a hazmat suit to try and talk me into staying in the hospital. I refused. When I left my room in a wheelchair, the nurses lined the hallway and cheered that the grumpy old man was leaving.

When we reached home, nobody there was happy. Sherrie and Jennifer thought I was being stubborn by refusing to stay in the hospital. I told them I was dying from Covid and renal failure, and I wasn't going to die alone in that hospital. I wanted to be with them.

Since it was Sunday, Dr. Gowda had no idea I had left the hospital. Sherrie wanted me to at least talk to Dr. Gowda again before we called hospice. I agreed. On Monday, Sherrie, Jennifer, and I had a Zoom call with Dr. Gowda. She was quite direct and went straight to the point.

"Mr. White," she said, "it's really a very simple choice—it's either dialysis or death. You need to discuss this with your family and make a decision. Call me tomorrow and let me know what you decide. If you choose dialysis, I will get you a chair time as quickly as I can. If you choose hospice, I can suggest a few locations."

We all thanked her and hung up. My house was quiet for a long while after that.

At that point, Dr. Gowda knew I was in a very fragile state of mind. She wasn't sure what I would do, but she was optimistic that Sherrie and Jennifer would convince me to try dialysis again.

Jennifer and Sherrie were clearly in the dialysis camp. I wasn't the least bit sure. My poor experience with dialysis in the hospital loomed very large in my mind, and Sherrie and Jennifer had absolutely no visibility into that experience. They were asking me to sign up for something that they knew nothing about.

There is no bigger decision a person can make than choosing between life and death. This decision was mine alone to make, and I had to make it very soon.

I decided to pray. "Lord, You told me You had this, and now I have Covid. I'm really ready to come home. I trust You to tell me what You want me to do, and when I know it is from You, I will do it."

The next day I felt as if God were saying, "I do have your health. Don't worry about that. You know I am faithful. But you have unfinished business with our book, and you need to finish that work." That's when I decided to give dialysis one more try.

Dr. Gowda then set me up for my first dialysis treatment at the Pure Life Renal Dialysis Clinic. I was not looking forward to it.

Takeaways

1. My Covid experience brought out the worst in me. I was ashamed of my behavior. I confessed this to God and asked that my focus return to Him. Don't let this happen to you. Everyone was trying their best to help me, but I didn't appreciate it. *We are not in control of what happens to us, but we are in control of we think about it.* I temporarily lost my focus, and I'll never do that again.

2. *When faced with life-or-death decisions, you need something to live for to choose life.* Maybe it's children, or grandchildren, or a mission or goal you have left to do in this life. Find your reason to live and fight for it. Never let go!

3. *If you choose death, make sure that you know Jesus first.*

9

Dialysis

I showed up at the Pure Life Renal Dialysis Clinic at 1:00 p.m. on Monday, February 1, 2021. I was in terrible shape. I was still suffering from many COVID-19 side effects including low oxygen levels, trouble breathing, Afib, using a walker (with help), and still no taste or smell. I had no fever and I don't know if I was contagious or not, but probably not since they were treating me. We were all masked, six feet apart, and the nurses wore hazmat suits.

The clinic's facility administrator is a nurse named Tonya Rolle. The procedure when you enter the clinic is that they take your temperature and weigh you. I needed help getting from the car into the clinic, but then Tonya took over. Sherrie and Jennifer were told to pick me up in four hours. I finally arrived at my chair, and they took my blood pressure. Then Tonya began to prepare the needles for insertion into my arm.

I was nervous because I knew how the pain was going to feel. But to my surprise, it was nothing like the pain I had experienced in the hospital. Now don't get me wrong, it was not pain-free, but it was nothing like before.

I later interviewed Tonya for this book, and I asked her what Dr. Gowda had told her about me and how she had been advised to treat me. Tonya said, "Dr. Gowda told me you were sick, and that you were considering hospice, but you were giving dialysis one more try." She told Dr. Gowda that the treatment went well, that I did well, but she wasn't sure I'd come back. But I did! Tonya told me later, "You looked really bad to me, and I wasn't sure you were going to continue with it."

A few treatments later, I was at least getting used to the routine. I would go in at 1:00 and leave at 5:00 p.m. The needles still hurt, but at least I knew what to expect. By this time, Tonya knew that I had a good support system in my wife and daughter. She knew this is critical for patients to stay on dialysis long-term.

Some pictures below of dialysis:

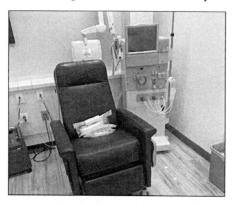

A typical dialysis chair next to the dialysis machine, which filters your blood.

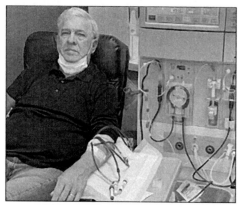

This is me in the chair during a dialysis treatment.

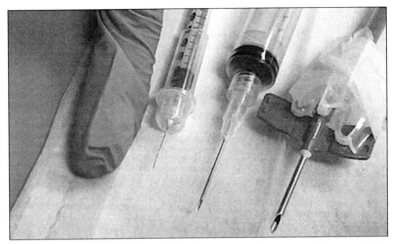

A series of needles. At the left is the nurse's finger, the first needle is for typical inoculations, next is a typical needle for drawing blood, and the last needle is the large one they use for dialysis.

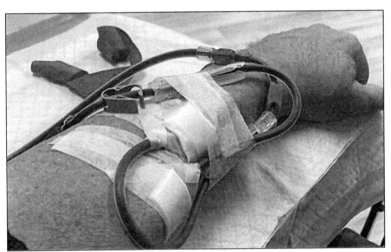

This is my arm during a dialysis treatment. One tube takes the blood out, and the other puts it back after cleaning.

Tonya is a very experienced dialysis nurse with almost forty years of experience. She has three grown children who all live in Florida. The saddest part for me is that Tonya is leaving at the end of the year. I will miss her. She has become the "face of dialysis" for me. When I hear the word dialysis, I see her face. She promised to keep in touch, and I'm going to hold her to that.

For Tonya, nursing has never been about the money. She has a passion for helping people. Her greatest asset is that she takes ownership of whatever responsibility she is given. I asked her what was the hardest part of dialysis nursing and she said, "It is getting patients to comply and do the things they are told." Her best advice to patients is to watch your diet (foods to eat and not eat), watch your fluids (only thirty-two ounces per day), don't ever skip a treatment, and use the ball regularly. The ball is provided by the vascular surgeon after the fistula is created. It fits in the palm of your hand, and squeezing it helps the fistula mature.

The Dialysis Treatment Regimen

I have dialysis three days each week (Monday, Wednesday, and Friday) and my treatment time is four hours. This is typical but varies by patient.

When I enter the clinic, the first thing they do is take my temperature and give me a mask. The next thing they do is weigh me. Weight is a critical measurement and determines how much fluid they will remove from you during your treatment. They weigh you again after your treatment when you leave. The difference between your exit weight on Wednesday and your entry weight on Friday tells the nurses how much fluid you have put on and is the primary driver for how much fluid they try to take off.

They refer to your normal weight as your dry weight or your exit weight. When your dry weight changes through diet or other reasons, they can adjust your dry weight to get a more accurate reading of your pure fluid gain.

Normally for me, they take off anywhere from 1.5 liters to 2.5 liters of fluid. The most they have taken from me was 3.5 liters, over a weekend where I didn't pay much attention to fluid intake (32 ounces per day is the guideline). When they take off too much fluid, I usually begin to cramp. For me it is usually my feet and calves, but it can affect the thighs as well. The nurse can stop the fluid removal when you cramp.

Removing 3.5 liters of fluid is more than you think. Imagine a two-liter bottle of soda on the grocery store shelf. It is a lot of fluid.

After weigh-in, I wash my fistula with soapy water and go to my chair. Once at my chair they take my standing BP. They leave the cuff on your arm the entire treatment time, and the machine automatically takes your BP every thirty minutes for the duration. After this it is time for the needles, which is the worst part of the process for me.

The needle that removes my blood goes in facing my wrist, and the needle that puts my cleansed blood back in my body goes in facing my elbow. For me, my "clearance" is best when the needle tips are as far apart as possible. Clearance is a term used to measure the cleanliness of your blood before dialysis and after dialysis. Once a month they draw blood before and after treatment to determine your clearance.

Let me just say something about these needles. They are big (see the pictures). These are fourteen-gauge needles. When removed they leave a scab. A normal needle to draw blood bleeds a little, then you can't see where it went in anymore.

With a dialysis needle you can see the scab! After the needles are in, they add a syringe of Heparin, which is a blood thinner that keeps the blood from clotting. After five minutes, they connect my needles to the hoses that are connected to the machine. My blood flows through the machine where it is cleansed via a filter, fluid is also extracted at the appropriate level, and the blood is returned back into my body through the other needle.

One of the reasons that fluid is such an important factor is because, over time, your kidneys cease to produce urine and fill your bladder, and you therefore cease most urination. When you don't eliminate fluid through urine, it must be eliminated through the dialysis process. This is also a big reason why they don't ever want you to skip treatments.

There is also something called infiltration. This is when the needle goes into the vein but punctures the other side and comes out in your arm. This is no fun and it has happened to me several times, all of which were my fault. You have to keep your arm very still. The needles are not catheter-like and flexible like many regular needles. They are steel and don't bend. If you move your arm, they can go all the way through your vein. I fell asleep once during dialysis, my arm moved in my sleep, and the needle went through the vein.

The specific needle was the one putting my blood back in my body, except now it was putting that blood into my arm, not the vein. Quickly a nurse came over and clamped off the tube, which stopped the blood flow. Then they had to insert a new needle in to finish giving me back the rest of my blood. They put cold compresses on my arm to stop any internal bleeding. My arm turned black and blue, and it took over a month to clear up.

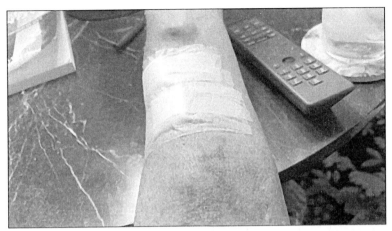

This is what happens with infiltration, when the needle goes all the way through your vein. The blood then flows into your arm causing the bruising. The arm is very swollen.

Another thing that they do on a monthly basis is draw blood for a complete blood chemistry workup. A nutritionist brings me my results every month and goes over them with me. They specifically measure protein, calcium, phosphorus, potassium, hemoglobin, and creatinine. She tells me what foods cause my numbers to go up or down. I usually hear, "Eat more of this and eat less of that."

When my four hours are completed, they remove the needles. Because the needles are so big, you must apply pressure for five minutes or so and then wear the bandages for several more hours before removing them. They take my BP—both seated and standing—take my temperature again, and then weigh me.

My treatments are now very early. I must be there at 5:15 a.m., and I'm in the chair from 5:30–9:30 a.m. I am usually home by 10:00 a.m. I'm not a good sleeper so I'm usually up early anyway, and this gives me all the rest of the day.

People always ask me, "What do you do for four hours?" Well, each chair is equipped with a television, or you can read, use your phone, iPad, or computer, or you can sleep.

Traveling on dialysis requires planning. I have done some traveling that required me to use another dialysis facility. Usually DaVita has multiple treatment locations in most major cities. I have found them to be very similar to my dialysis facility and the process to be equally similar. It pays to know your typical fluid removal levels and any special needling instructions.

The secretary in my clinic is named Judy, and she makes all my travel arrangements for dialysis. I give her the address of where I'll be staying, and she finds the closet dialysis clinic and makes all the arrangements. She sends all my dialysis medical information, gets the dates for treatments, and my chair time on those days. Judy really makes it easy for me.

My biggest adjustment to dialysis was how it became my whole life. It seemed as though I was either getting ready for dialysis, having dialysis, or recovering from dialysis. It seemed to consume me, and I forgot that I had a life outside of dialysis. I had to work really hard at continuing to do all the other things that I enjoyed. It took me several months to break out of that funk.

Now I look at dialysis as my part-time job. Before I retired, I worked forty to fifty hours every week. Now I have a part-time job that is only three days per week and only four hours a day. When I'm at dialysis, I don't have to do anything!

Takeaways

1. *Don't let dialysis become your life.* Keep doing all the things you used to do. Go to the movies, go out to dinner, have picnics, take walks. Just stay occupied with life, not dialysis.

2. *My faith and trust in God have been essential for me.* Read the gospel of John and earnestly ask God to reveal Himself to you.

   Ask and it will be given to you; seek and you will find; knock and the door will be opened for you. For everyone who asks receives; the one who seeks finds; and to the one who knocks, the door will be opened (Matt. 7:7-8).

   Test God on this!

10

The Journey Continues

When I left the hospital in early February, I had Afib. My doctors thought COVID-19 was the cause and that when I got over the virus, my Afib would go away too. No such luck! I went to see my cardiologist, Dr. Laura Gonzalez. She wanted to be very proactive in getting rid of it and so did I.

The first approach she wanted to try was the least invasive, a cardioversion. Basically, they put you to sleep with a little Propofol, and they zap you with the paddles as you see on TV. Many times this will shock the heart back into normal rhythm. It worked for me on the first jolt.

If the cardioversion had not gotten my heart back in rhythm, then they would have used other rhythmic medications in addition to Eliquis®. If Afib persisted, then they would move forward with an ablation, which involves going through the groin and up to the heart to do some magic with radiofrequency. Of course, if a patient has no symptoms from Afib, her or she could remain on blood thinners forever and live with the Afib.

One danger with Afib is that it tends to throw off blood clots, so most often they put you on blood thinners. They put me on Eliquis®, which was over $300 per month, so I was anxious to get rid of it. They could have put me on other blood thinners, like Coumadin, but Dr. Gonzalez was limited in the drugs she could use because of my renal disease. Also, Eliquis® has a better track record in preventing strokes. Dr. Gonzalez wanted me to stay on the Eliquis® for another six months, so I had no better choice.

For the last thirty days Dr. Gonzalez had me on a heart monitor. The monitor showed I had no episodes of Afib over that timeframe, and I was finally able to get off the blood thinners. I will continue to see Dr. Gonzalez every six months or so.

Another thing that happened in April 2021 was I reached out to Urologist Brendon Fels, who had diagnosed my renal cell carcinoma. Brendon had recommended to the transplant team that they move forward and give me the new kidney. While the transplant team had accepted his recommendation, they also planned to remove the renal cell kidney about one month after the transplant. Since I didn't have the transplant, or the surgery to remove the renal cell carcinoma, I still had that cancer inside me, and I wanted to see what he recommended we do about it.

He recommended another MRI to see if, and how much, it had grown. The results showed that the renal cell carcinoma was the exact same size. "Brendon," I asked, "wouldn't you have expected this to have grown some in a year's time? Are you sure this is really cancer?"

He began to question if it was cancer after all. However, he did say that carcinomas like this grow very slowly. He agreed to do another MRI in April 2022. If the results still show no growth, he will be willing to say one of two things: either it's not cancer, or it is so slow growing that it will never present a threat to me. We can then quit doing MRIs, and I'm good with that.

The summer of 2021 went by pretty quickly. We visited my brother in Annapolis for a week, and I went to a DaVita dialysis center. It proved to be a very similar experience to my dialysis at Pure Life Renal.

In September, I spoke to Dr. Gowda, who was doing her rounds at the clinic, about my blood work and my general health. We chatted a bit. She knew I was an author, and she suggested I write this book. She said she thought there was a great need for a book like this that told a story and shared the experiences and choices that patients face. I prayed about it, and it just felt as if God was behind it. That's when I started to write, and all my doctors agreed to be interviewed for the book.

Takeaways

1. *Follow up with all your doctors on a regular basis.* When something doesn't feel right, or if you have questions, go see them. Always remember that bad news early is good news!

2. *You need God every day,* even for the routine moments of life.

11

Testing Comparisons

The social worker at my dialysis clinic asked me to participate in a survey that has been used with thousands of other dialysis patients nationwide. With no right or wrong answers, it's just a measurement of how you feel about your experience. It measured five key areas and compared my score to the nationwide average (over 10,000 people). It compared me to my peers (male, about my age, and without diabetes). It then gave suggestions for how to improve one's score in each category.

The five categories were:

1. **Physical Component Summary** (PCS): This reports how you feel about your physical health. In the survey you are asked if you could do things like climb stairs, move a table, or push a vacuum. How well you think you feel physically is a key measure to your health. With all other things being equal, the PCS score predicts who would not need hospital care and who was likely to live longer. The average score in this category was 35.4%. Some steps you can take to improve your score are:

- Be more active.

- Exercise.

- Keep your hemoglobin in the target range.

- Eat more protein.

- Eat less salt to keep fluid weight down.

2. **Mental Component Summary** (MCS): This reports how you feel about your mental and emotional health. In the survey you are asked about whether you felt calm, had enough energy, or felt blue. The MCS score predicts who might need a hospital stay and who was likely to live longer. The average score in this category was 45.5%. Some measures you can take to improve your score are:

- Believe that you can have a good life.

- Do things you love.

- Keep enjoying your hobbies.

- Challenge yourself.

- Connect with others.

- Make choices about your future.

3. **Burden of Kidney Disease**: This score measures your feelings about how much kidney disease affects your life. In the survey you are asked if kidney disease takes up too much time, frustrates you, or makes you feel like a burden to family or others. The average score in this category was 41.6%. Some ways you can improve your score are:

- Do what you can for yourself.

- Learn all you can about kidney disease and treatment.

- Make good use of your treatment time.

- Look into other dialysis treatment options.

4. **Symptoms and Problems**: This score measures how much you feel bothered by day-to-day symptoms or problems

caused by dialysis. In the survey you are asked about chest pain, cramps, itching, and shortness of breath, loss of appetite, upset stomach, feeling washed out, and other symptoms. The average score in this category was 72.6%. Some actions you can take to improve your score are:

- Follow your treatment plan.
- Know your fluid goal.
- Get enough dialysis.
- Baby your skin.
- Care for your dialysis access.
- Report new symptoms.

5. **Effects of Kidney Disease on Daily Life**: This score measures how much impact kidney disease has on your day. In the survey you are asked about fluid and diet limits and how well you think you can work around the house and travel. This section also asks about stress, how dependent you feel on doctors, your sex life, and your appearance. The average score in this category was 72.6%. To improve your score, you can do the following:

- Get more dialysis.
- Keep moving.
- Put in your own needles.
- Keep your sense of humor.
- Communicate with your partner.
- Be realistic.

I recommend that any dialysis patient ask their social worker to administer this survey and provide you with your results. It gives you a great sense of how well you're doing compared to others.

Takeaways

1. *Find ways like the test above to measure yourself* against your peers. It is a comfort to know that you are doing as well as most people, and if not, to get some ideas of how to improve. Who knows, maybe your score will lead the pack, and you'll be the example for others.

12

Depression

I feel pretty good these days, but I did go see a psychiatrist recently, Dr. Wendy Baer, who was referred to me by my oncologist, Dr. Sarah Friend.

I have a history of depression. In fact, I was hospitalized with it about twenty-five years ago. I have been off the depression meds now for several years, but I felt as if I needed to get back on medication. Dr. Baer prescribed Bupropion 150mg XL, which I was on previously, and hopefully I will feel better soon.

When I was hospitalized earlier, I learned a lot about Cognitive Behavioral Therapy (CBT). In a book entitled *Feeling Good*, author Dr. David Burns describes ten typical distorted ways of thinking in depressed people. Because depressed people have a different way of thinking, you can examine your own thoughts (CBT) and know if you're slipping back into depression.

One of his examples is called "the perfectionist." If a perfectionist gets a 99% on a test, they think they have failed because their 99% didn't reach the perfect score of 100%. You can see that this is a distorted view of how they did on the test. In the book he describes nine other distorted types of thinking. If we can see ourselves thinking in one of these distorted ways, we can then self-correct our distorted thinking to combat the depression.

As you have read about my journey with kidney disease thus far, you can probably see why I might be depressed. Your journey might make you depressed as well.

Dr. Baer specializes in treating patients with cancer. Severe medical issues can easily lead to depression, and it's not unusual.

There is some stigma today in society about people suffering from mental illness. Certainly depression is a mental illness, but the stigma ought to be about people not getting treatment, not about having depression. It is a treatable illness.

Diabetics take insulin to control their illness so they can live a normal life. People with depression can get counseling and medication and also live a normal life. It is a small price to pay to be well.

Takeaways

1. *Don't hesitate to get help.* Depression is common in people with morbid diseases, and help is available. You're going through enough; don't let depression add to your condition!

13

The Kidney Project

The Kidney Project is a joint venture by the University of California San Francisco (UCSF) and Vanderbilt University. The purpose is to engineer an artificial kidney to be implanted in the patient to improve the lives of patients with renal failure. There are no pumps, tubes, immunosuppressant drugs, or dialysis.

Dr. Shuvo Roy from UCSF is the Project Director. He says, "The basic technology of hemodialysis has been unchanged since the early 1970s. We are changing the underlying technology of the artificial filters that separate wastes from blood. This allows us to miniaturize the filters so they can fit inside the human body. We allow the patient's own heart to circulate blood to the filters. Instead of requiring hundreds of gallons of water for dialysis, we use the body's own naturally-evolved biological strategy to concentrate wastes into one or two liters of urine."

They have made great progress to date, but funding remains a major challenge. Original forecasts were to have a human trial in 2020. As of the writing of this book, they have not received approval from the FDA to proceed with a human trial. I asked Dr. Gowda what she thought about the Kidney Project, and she said she thought it would be quite some time before human trials were approved, even longer for wide-scale use. She believes that one day it will happen, but her position now is just "wait and see."

I encourage everyone to learn more about The Kidney Project. They have a Facebook page that you can join to get regular updates on the project. You can also go to pharm.ucsf.edu or the Vanderbilt University website for more information. I have spoken to Dr. Roy on several occasions and exchanged many emails with him. His email address is shuvo.roy@ucsf.edu, and his telephone number is 415-514-9666.

Takeaways

1. *Medical breakthroughs happen all the time.* Someday artificial kidneys will be a reality, perhaps soon enough to benefit you. Stay informed about what is going on and what is being done in kidney disease. Never give up; there is always hope!

14

The Good News

At some point in our life we will all face our own mortality. Mine came during COVID-19 when my kidneys failed. What happens after we die? Where do we go? What will it be like? How can anyone know for sure? Most everyone would really like to know, so let me share a few of my thoughts.

I believe the Bible and I believe in heaven and hell. Many do; some don't. We can all admit that we have done some bad things in our life, wrong things, things we wish we could take back. We feel guilt about those areas, and we feel in some way that we should be punished for them. The Bible calls them sins.

Just like when we were punished as kids by our parents for our transgressions, God must punish our sins. In order to become righteous we must be forgiven, and that usually occurs after the punishment.

In the Old Testament the Israelites had the Ten Commandments and were taught to obey them. Their righteousness came from obeying the law. When they broke the law, they sacrificed animals on the altar as atonement for their sins.

God wanted to love His creation (mankind), but at the same time God had to be just and therefore punish sin. The punishment for sin is death! How could God love and punish sin at the same time?

God chose to become a man in the person of His Son,

Jesus Christ! Jesus was 100 percent man while being 100 percent God. God's grand idea was that Jesus would be the sacrifice needed for all mankind's sins. No more animal sacrifices every week but one sacrifice for all people for all time. His sinless Son was the only one who could fulfill God's grand idea. That is exactly what He did when he died on that cross on Calvary's hill.

Therefore, righteousness can come to us from God, not from obeying the law. God showed His love for mankind by providing His Son as a sacrifice, atoning for all mankind's sin. He was justified in doing so because sin had been paid for by the death of His Son.

Romans 3:21-26 says,

But now apart from the law the righteousness of God has been made known . . . This righteousness is given through faith in Jesus Christ to all who believe . . . all have sinned and fall short of the glory of God, and all are justified freely by His grace through the redemption that came by Christ Jesus. God presented Christ as a sacrifice of atonement, through the shedding of his blood—to be received by faith. He did this to demonstrate his righteousness . . . and the one who justifies those who have faith in Jesus.

How then does this righteousness from God come to us? By faith! By simply believing that Jesus died on the cross as atonement for our sins. And it is by God's grace that we are saved by faith. We don't work for it; we don't obey laws for it; we just accept it by faith. This is our salvation! On this faith hangs the answer to where you will spend eternity.

For God so loved the world that he gave his one and only Son, that whoever believes in him shall not perish but have eternal life (John 3:16).

Without such faith, the Bible teaches that people will spend eternity in hell.

My belief in this story of man's salvation has carried me through the trials and tribulations of the past three years. It truly has provided a peace that passes all understanding. The God who made provision for my salvation by sacrificing His Son as atonement for my sins has my absolute faith and trust for everything in my life.

Our salvation is a gift from God. Will you accept it?

Epilogue

At the time of this writing, it is now February 2022, and my medical condition is stable. I still do dialysis three times each week for four hours. My two cancers remain in observation mode, and the doctors are just waiting for me to become symptomatic.

Dr. Gowda attributes my great improvement since February to my attitude, careful dialysis treatment, and my compliance with all the doctors and nurses have asked me to do.

It seems like for almost three years now, it's been one thing after another. In the middle of it all, my coauthor, Joyce, sent me the following anonymous poem quoted by famous author Elizabeth Elliot, which has really helped me all along the way:

DO THE NEXT THING
At an old English parsonage down by the sea
There came in the twilight a message to me.
Its quaint Saxon legend deeply engraven
    that, as it seems to me, teaching from heaven.
And all through the hours the quiet words ring,
Like a low inspiration, DO THE NEXT THING.

Many a questioning, many a fear,
    many a doubt hath its quieting here.
Moment by moment, let down from heaven,
    time, opportunity, guidance is given.
Fear not tomorrow, child of the King
Trust that to Jesus, just DO THE NEXT THING.

Do it immediately, do it with prayer,
  do it reliantly, casting all care.
Do it with reverence, tracing His hand,
  who placed it before thee with earnest command.
Stayed on omnipotence, safe 'neath His wing,
Leave all the results, just DO THE NEXT THING.

Looking to Jesus, ever serener,
  working or suffering be thy demeanor
  in His dear presence, the rest of His calm,
  the light of His countenance, be thy psalm.
DO THE NEXT THING.

For the last three years I've just been doing the next thing, and I want you to do the next thing as well. Don't ever give up; just do the next thing.

What does the future hold for me? I know that I will probably not be a long-term dialysis patient because that is just not in my DNA. How long will I do dialysis? I just don't know. I have already skipped treatments just because I mentally needed a day off. This is probably not a good sign. I've talked to Sherrie about it, and she knows that I'm probably not in this for the long term.

I think the Lord will somehow let me know. I think the apostle Paul knew when he had finished his race, and I think I'll know too. Paul said,

The time for my departure is near. I have fought the good fight, I have finished the race, I have kept the faith (2 Tim. 4:6-7).

I'm trusting in God for that same knowledge. You know there are worse things than death. When you know you are going to heaven, it takes the entire sting away. I think of it as transitioning my care from my doctors to the Great Physician. As Paul said, "To live is Christ and to die is gain" (Phil. 1:21). Either way, I'm a winner!

I wish you the best of luck in your kidney disease journey. I hope what I've shared will help you. What helped me to this point was a good attitude about my situation and my close relationship with my heavenly Father. You trust your doctor, and you can trust the Great Physician! He is available to all of us!

Acknowledgments

Many people always play a significant role in the writing, editing, and publishing of a book. I must start with Dr. Anupama Gowda, my nephrologist, who has been with me since the day I was diagnosed with kidney disease. She has been professional and straightforward with me about my condition all along the way. I appreciate you, Dr. Gowda.

When I've asked all my other doctors if they know Dr. Gowda, the answer is always the same, "Oh, she is the best, one of the smartest doctors at Emory." Comments like that make a patient know they are in good hands. Dr. Gowda was the one who encouraged me to write this book because she felt there was a great need.

I also want to offer special thanks to Dr. Sarah Friend, my hematology oncologist. Dr. Friend was personally responsible for me getting cleared to receive a kidney transplant. She argued with the transplant team and successfully defended her recommendation to get me a new kidney. My other doctors think she is the best in her field. My friendship with Dr. Friend has been a bonus. You even read all my books! You're the best, Doc!

And thanks to my cardiologist, Dr. Laura Gonzales, who treated me for my Afib, which I got during COVID-19. She performed the cardioversion (zapping me with the paddles) that set my heart back in rhythm. After six months and wearing a heart monitor for thirty days, she finally took me off the blood thinners (Eliquis®).

All three of these fine doctors were interviewed for this book. I thank them all for their time and willingness to participate.

I also interviewed my dialysis nurse, Tonya Rolle. I see

Tonya now three days every week, and she is just a pleasure to be around. I dedicated this book to her.

Denise Neal was my transplant coordinator. She met with me for over two hours on a Sunday afternoon to be interviewed. I learned so much from her about the issues and concerns of the transplant team. Hats off to you, Denise. Denise and I are both big Georgia Bulldog football fans, and we worked hard to bring home that National Championship Trophy! Go Dawgs!

Also, I want give a big shout-out to Joyce and Peter Hill. Joyce coauthored my last book with me and helped in editing this one. Thank you, guys!

Also my publisher and editor, Brian and Kathy Banashak, at River Birch Press deserve a huge thank you for all their hard work in getting this book published.

And next to last, but not least, I want to thank my wife, Sherrie, for all her support. You are the love of my life and my best friend. I cherish you!

And no acknowledgment would be complete for me without thanking the good Lord. My Lord and Savior Jesus Christ has been with me through this whole ordeal, including the writing of this book. All of my trust and hope for the future is in Him.

My citizenship is in heaven, and I'll be home soon!

About the Author

STEVE WHITE is a retired management consultant. He has written books on psychology, parenting, and knowing God. He attends Northpoint Community Church. He is also a frequent speaker and educator. He has four children, eight grandchildren, and two great-grandchildren. He lives in Atlanta, Georgia, with his wife, Sherrie.